AF730638

NEUROSURGERY

for kids

Medical School
FOR KIDS™

Copyright © 2024 Betty Nguyen & Brandon Pham

All rights reserved. No part of this book may be reproduced or used in any manner without the prior written permission of the copyright owner, except for the use of brief quotations in a book review.

First paperback edition March 2024

Book design by Betty Nguyen & Brandon Pham

ISBN 978-1-957557-25-0 (paperback)

Printed in the United States of America

Published by Black Phoenix Press

www.mdforkids.org

Disclaimer: Contents of this book are for informational purposes only. No material in this book is intended to provide, or be a substitute for, professional medical advice.

To the friends and family who have supported and loved us unconditionally, and to the mentors who have guided and taught us more than we could have imagined:

Thank you.

Betty & Brandon

Medical School FOR KIDS™

Neurosurgery

(NUR-ow-sur-jr-ee)

the branch of medicine concerned with the diagnosis and surgical treatment of the nervous system, including the brain and spinal cord

Medical School FOR KIDS™

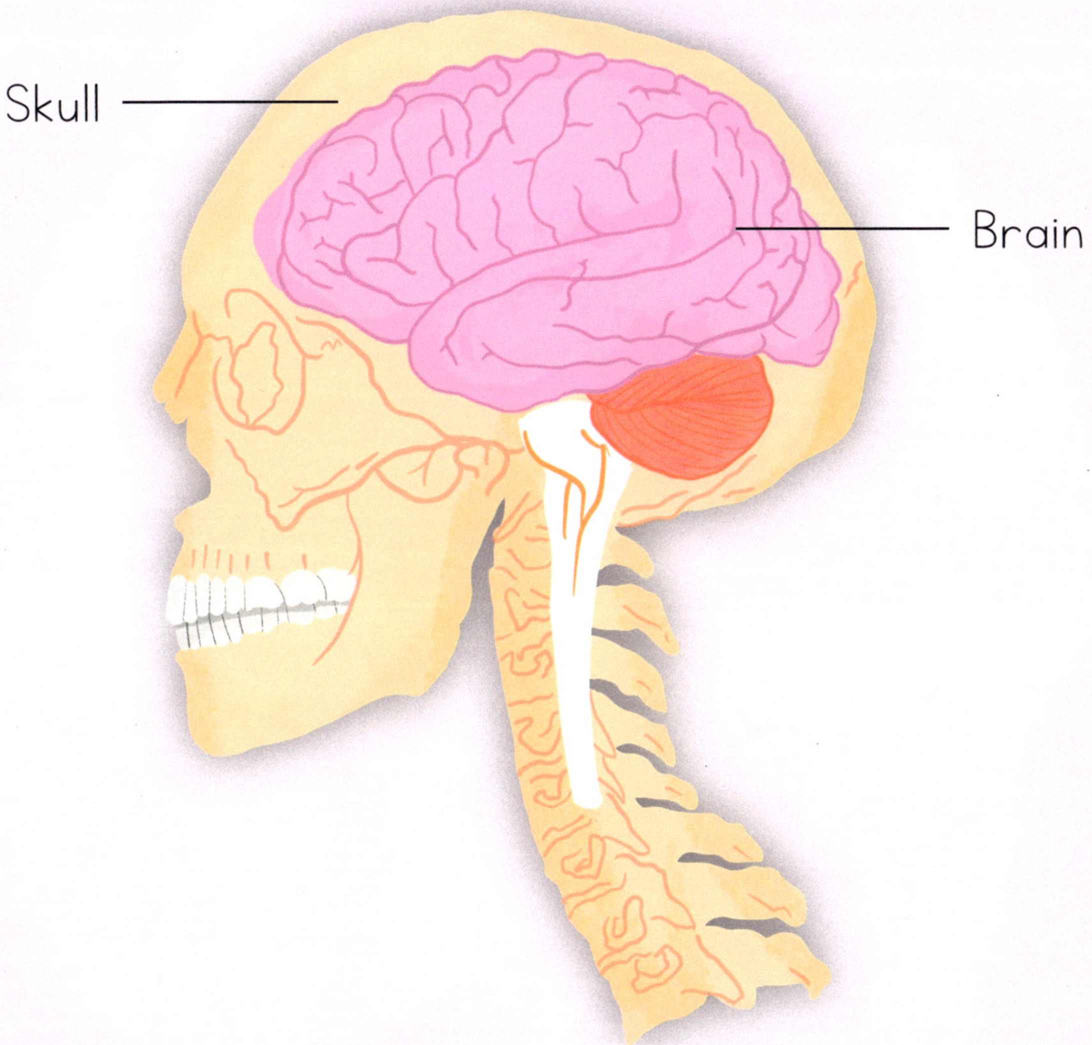

The **brain** is a pink and squishy organ in our head that allows us to think. A set of bones, called the **skull**, surrounds and protects our brain.

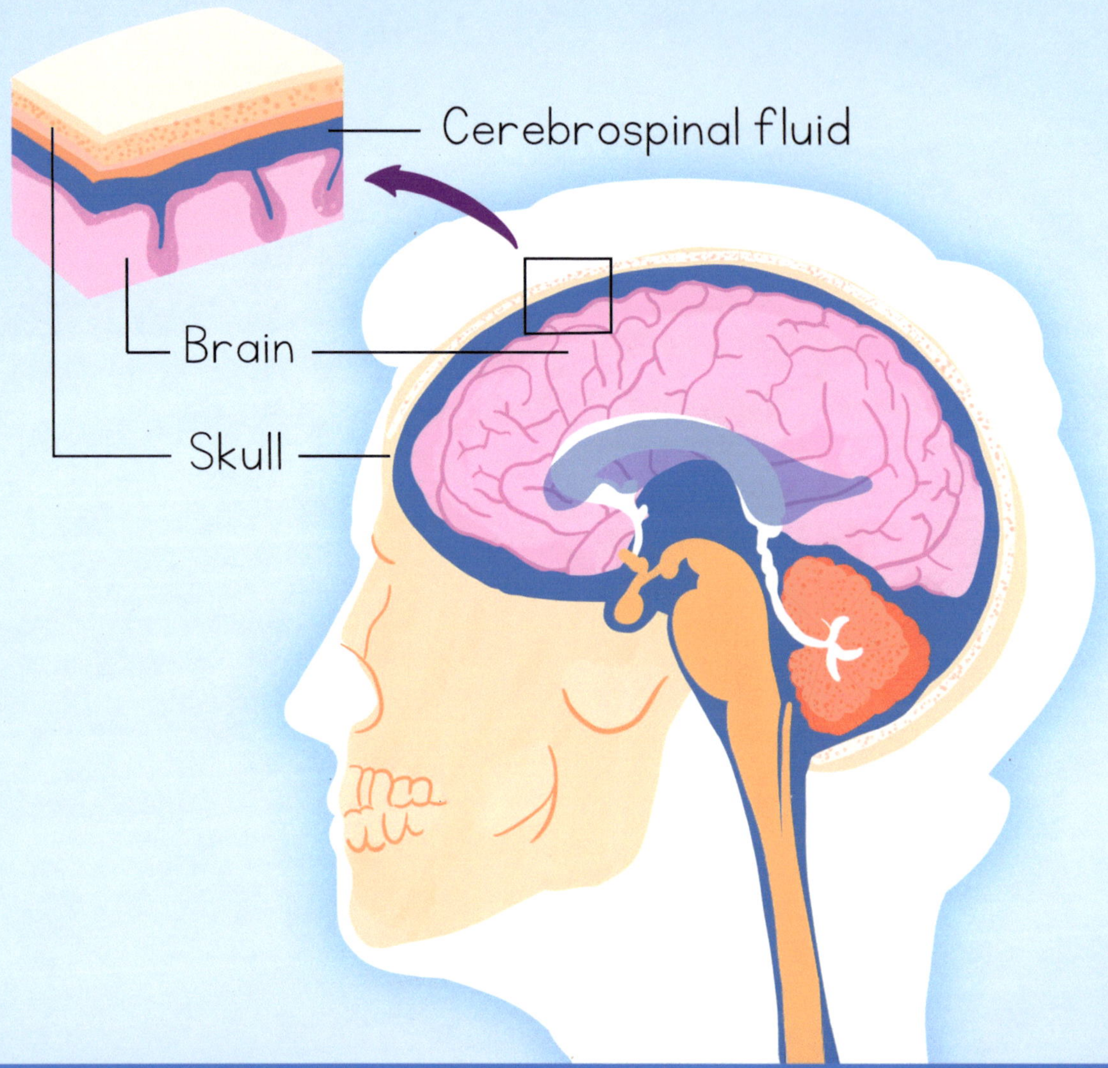

Our brain makes a special liquid called **cerebrospinal fluid** that cushions the brain and allows it to float in our skull.

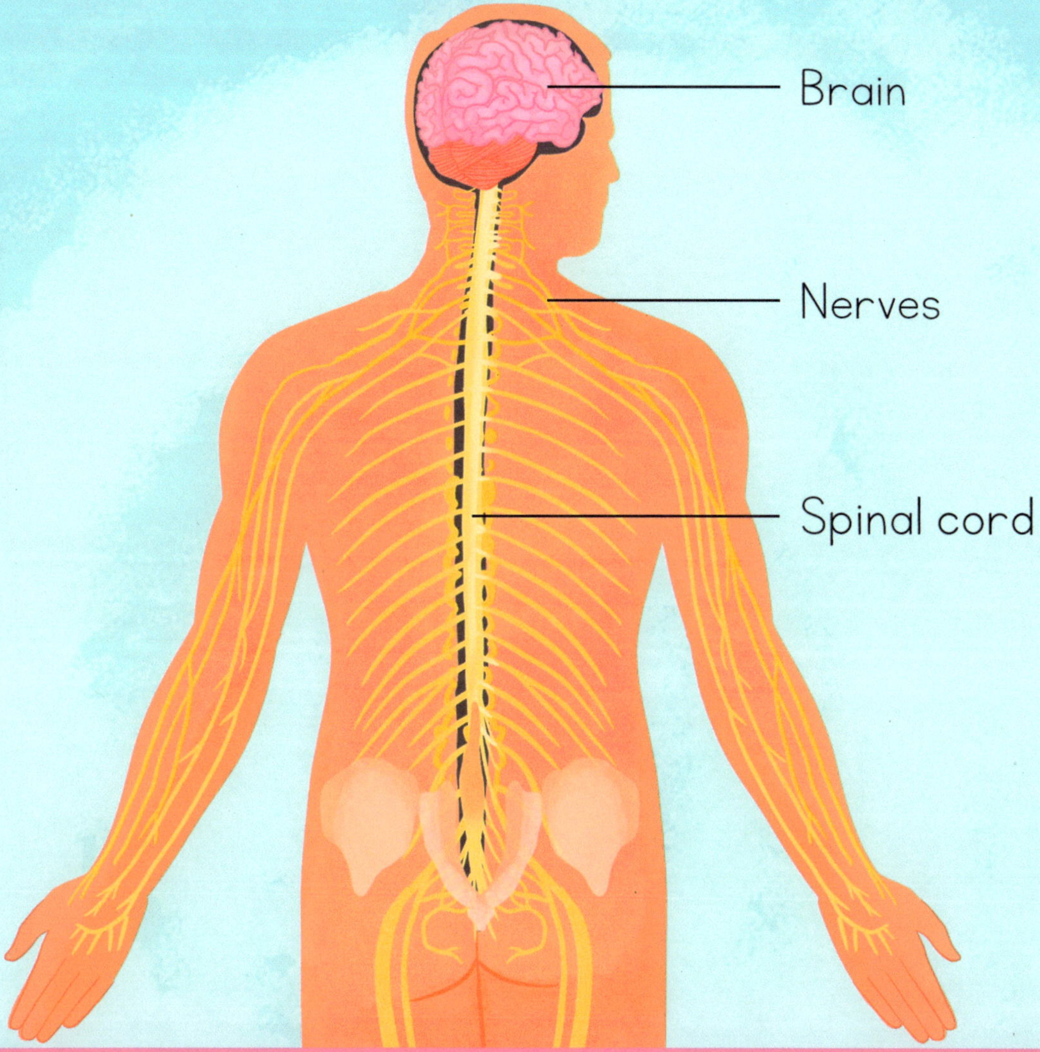

The **spinal cord** connects our brain to the rest of our body with **nerves** that branch out. This allows us to feel sensations and move our muscles.

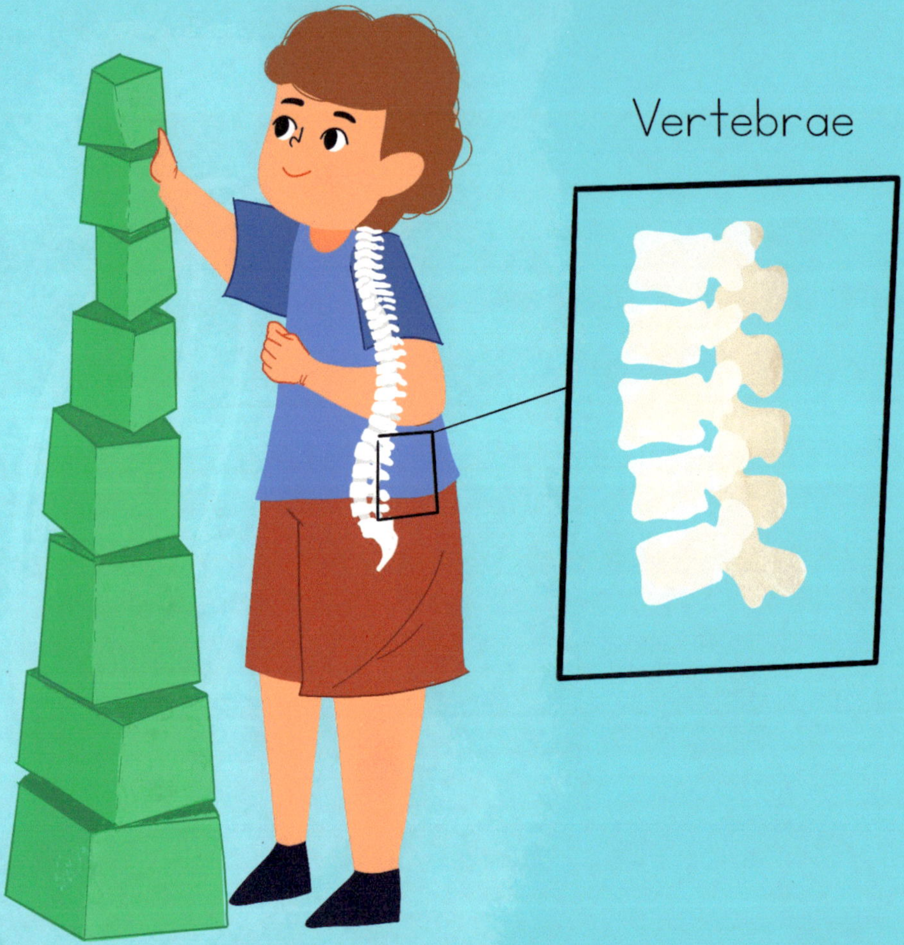

A stack of bones called **vertebrae** surrounds and protects our spinal cord and makes up our **spine**.

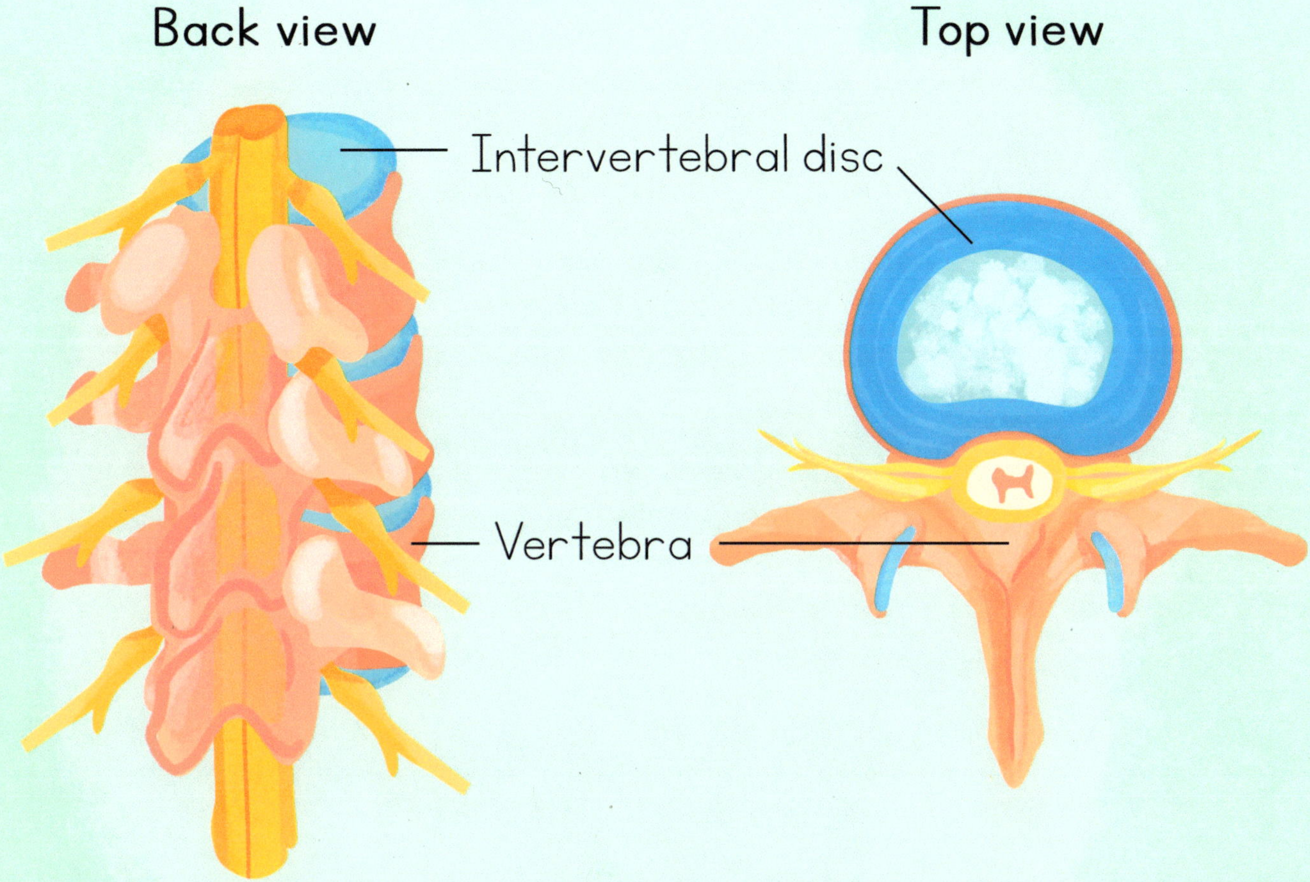

Between each vertebra is a cushion called an **intervertebral disc**, which allows movement and absorbs shock.

X-ray CT scan MRI scan

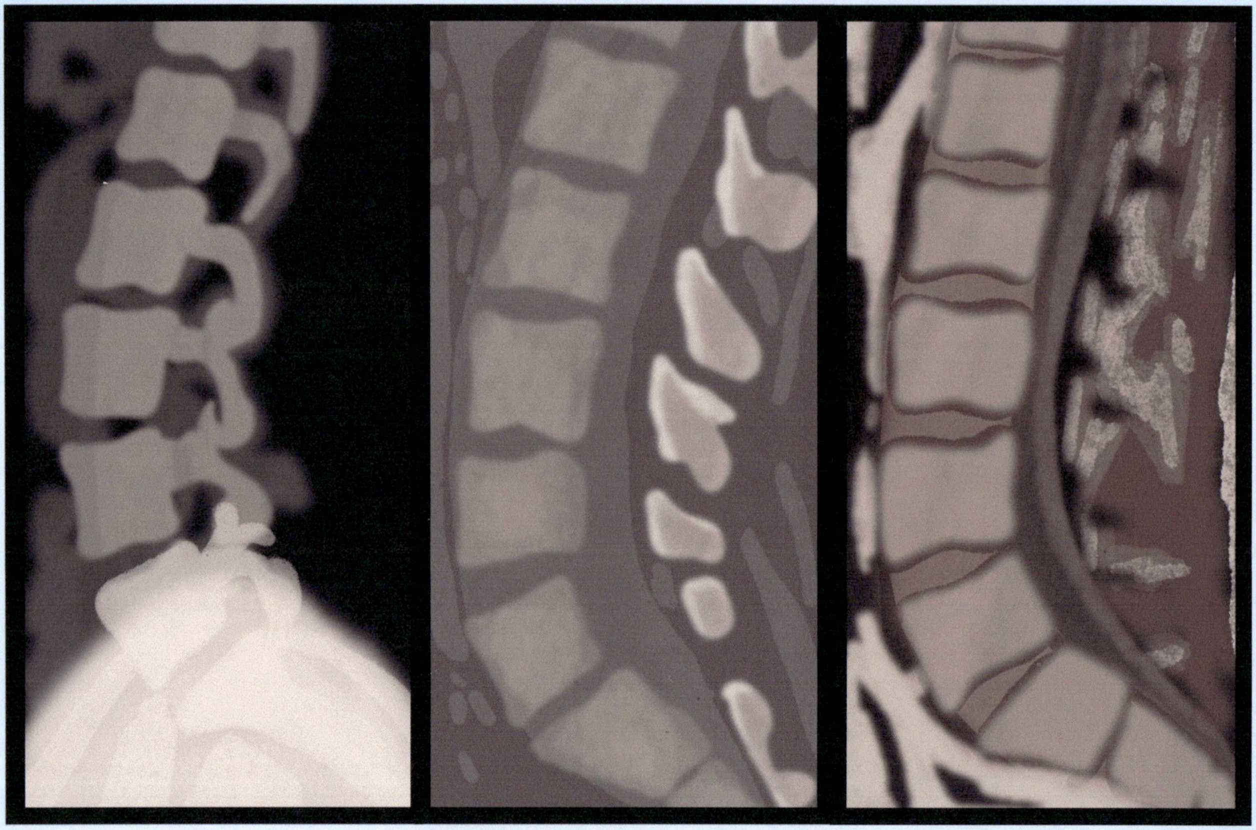

Doctors use imaging tests, such as X-rays, CT scans, and MRI scans, to diagnose problems that may occur in our brain, spine, and spinal cord.

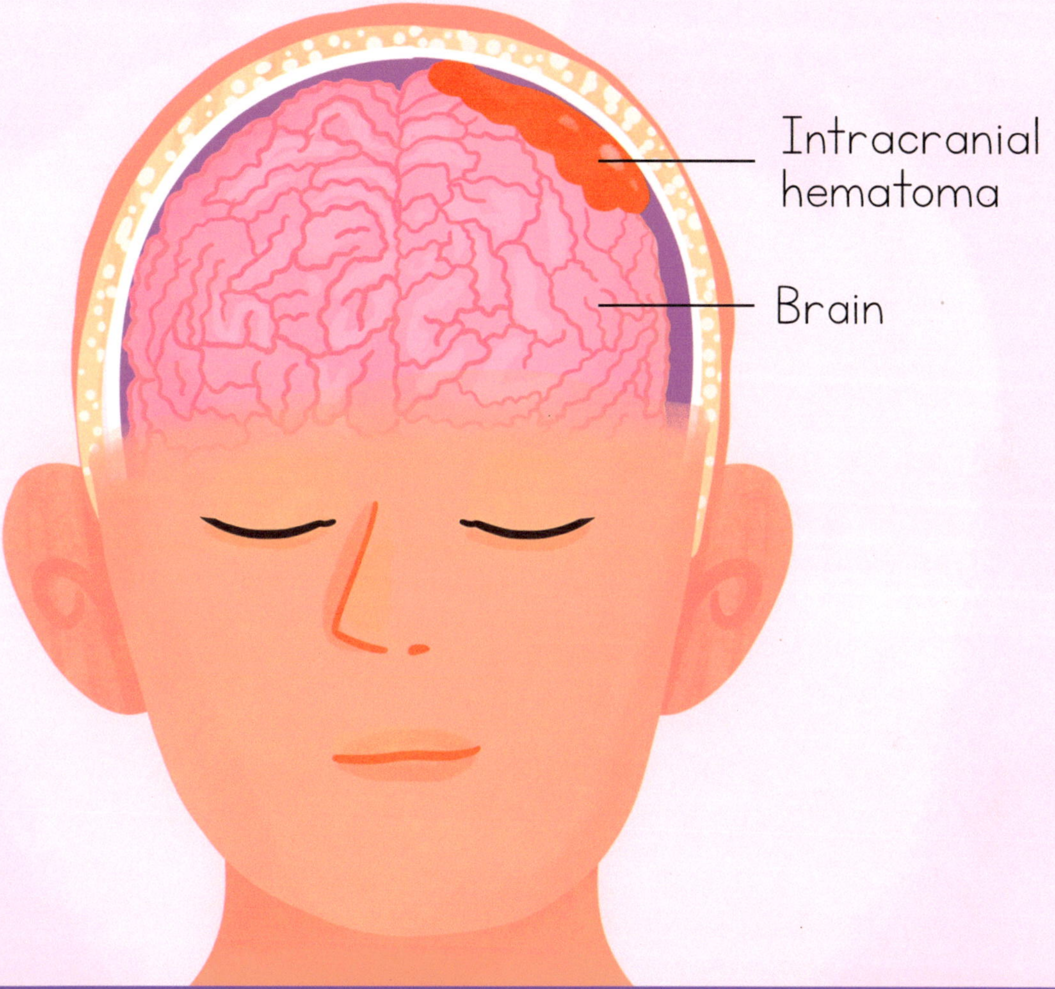

Sometimes, a big accident can injure the brain. If the blood vessels rupture, blood can leak out into the brain. This is called an **intracranial hematoma**.

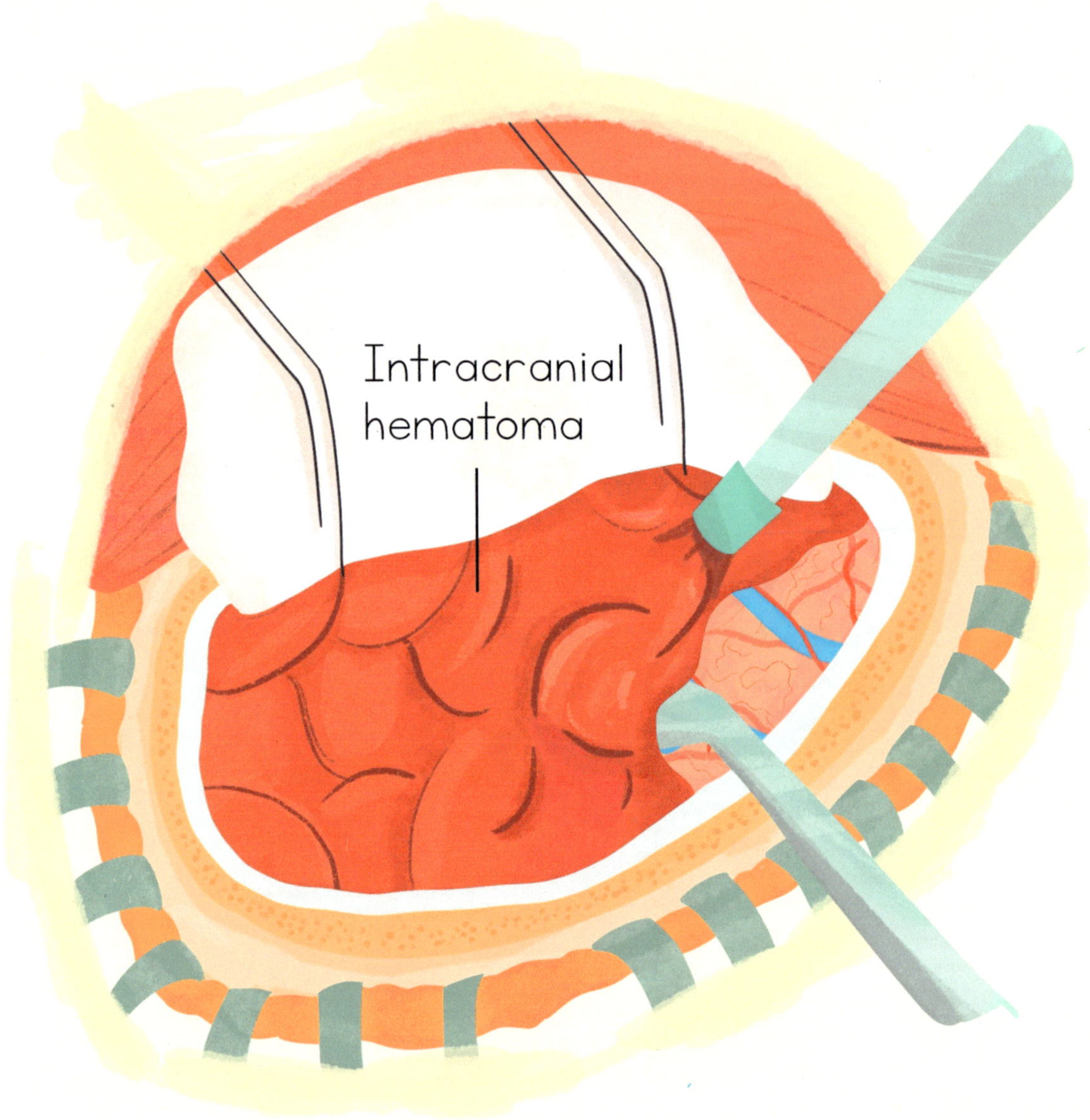

If severe enough, a surgery called a **craniotomy** can be done to remove the intracranial hematoma through a temporary opening in the skull.

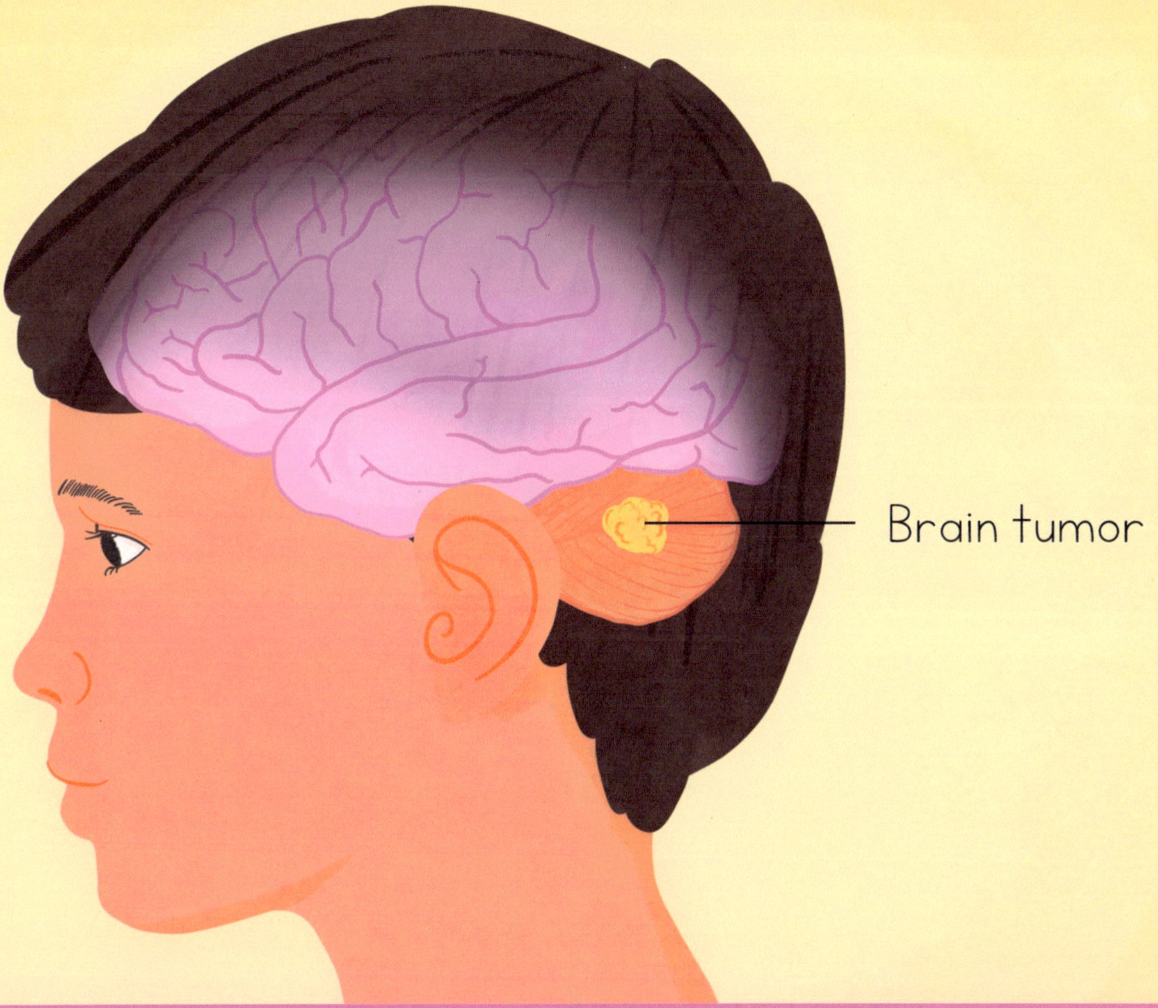

A **brain tumor** is an abnormal growth of cells in or around the brain. There are many types of brain tumors.

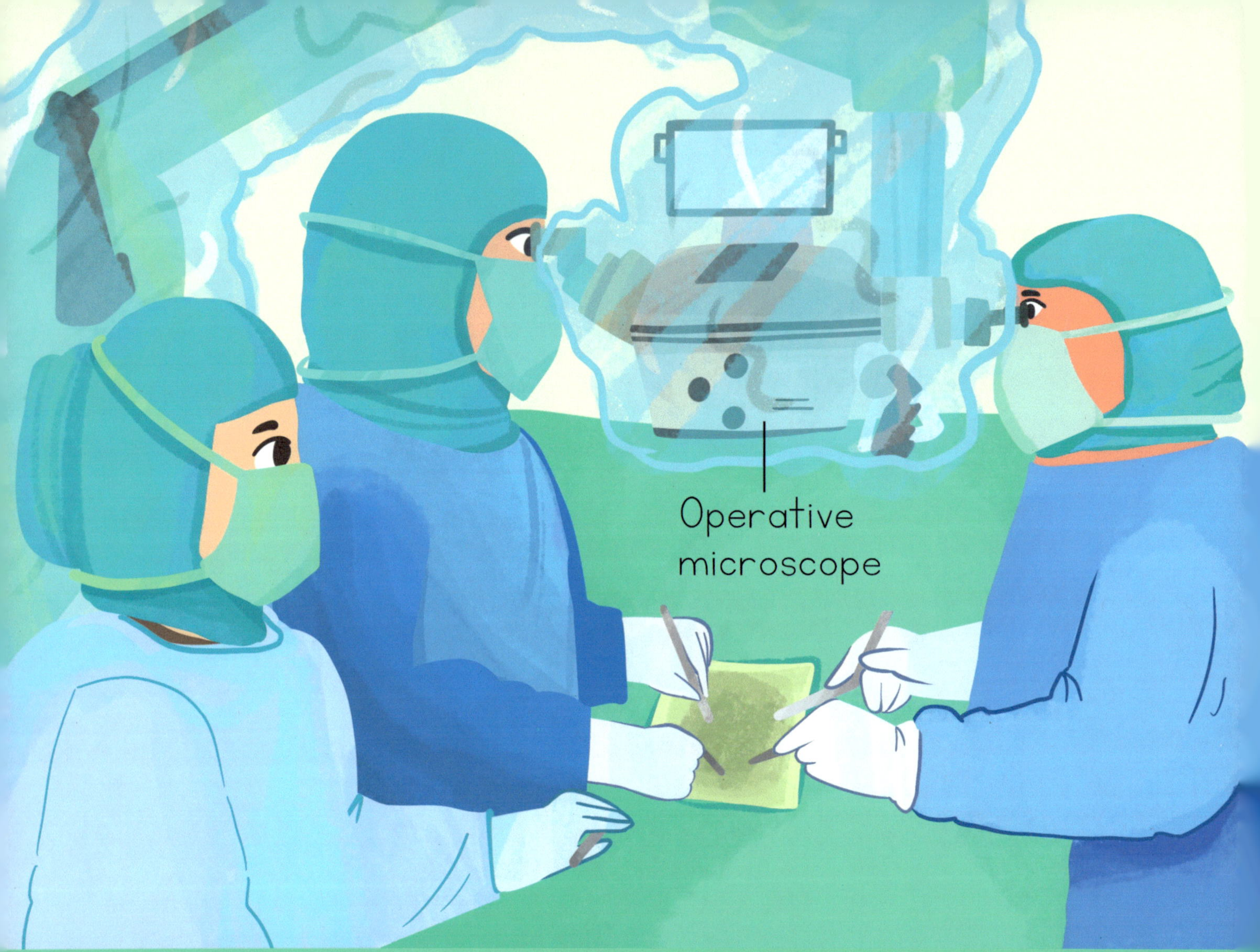

Neurosurgeons use an **operative microscope** to see tiny details in brain tissue and safely remove these tumors using small delicate tools.

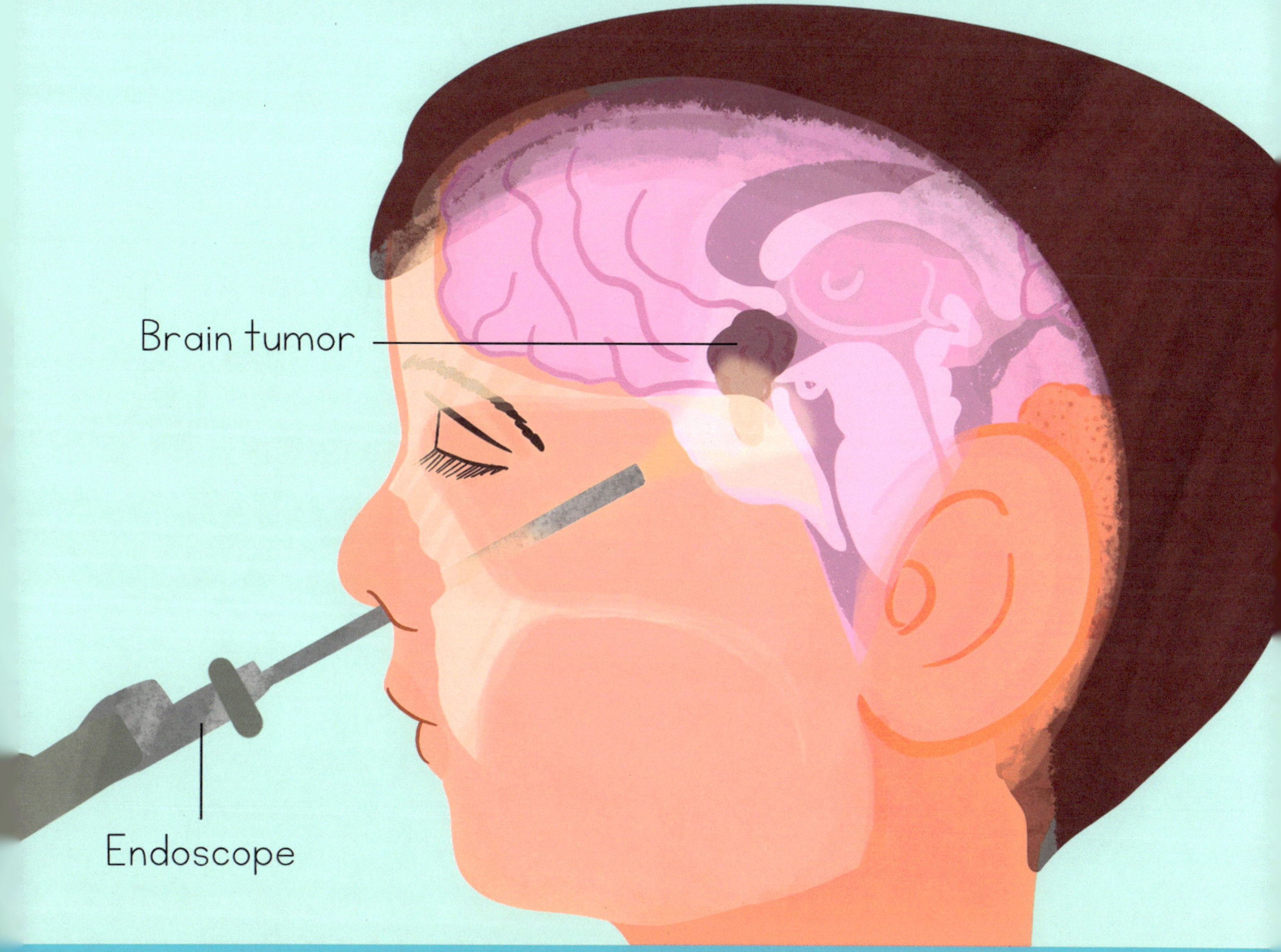

Some tumors that grow at the bottom of the skull, called the skull base, can be removed through the nose using a special camera called an **endoscope**.

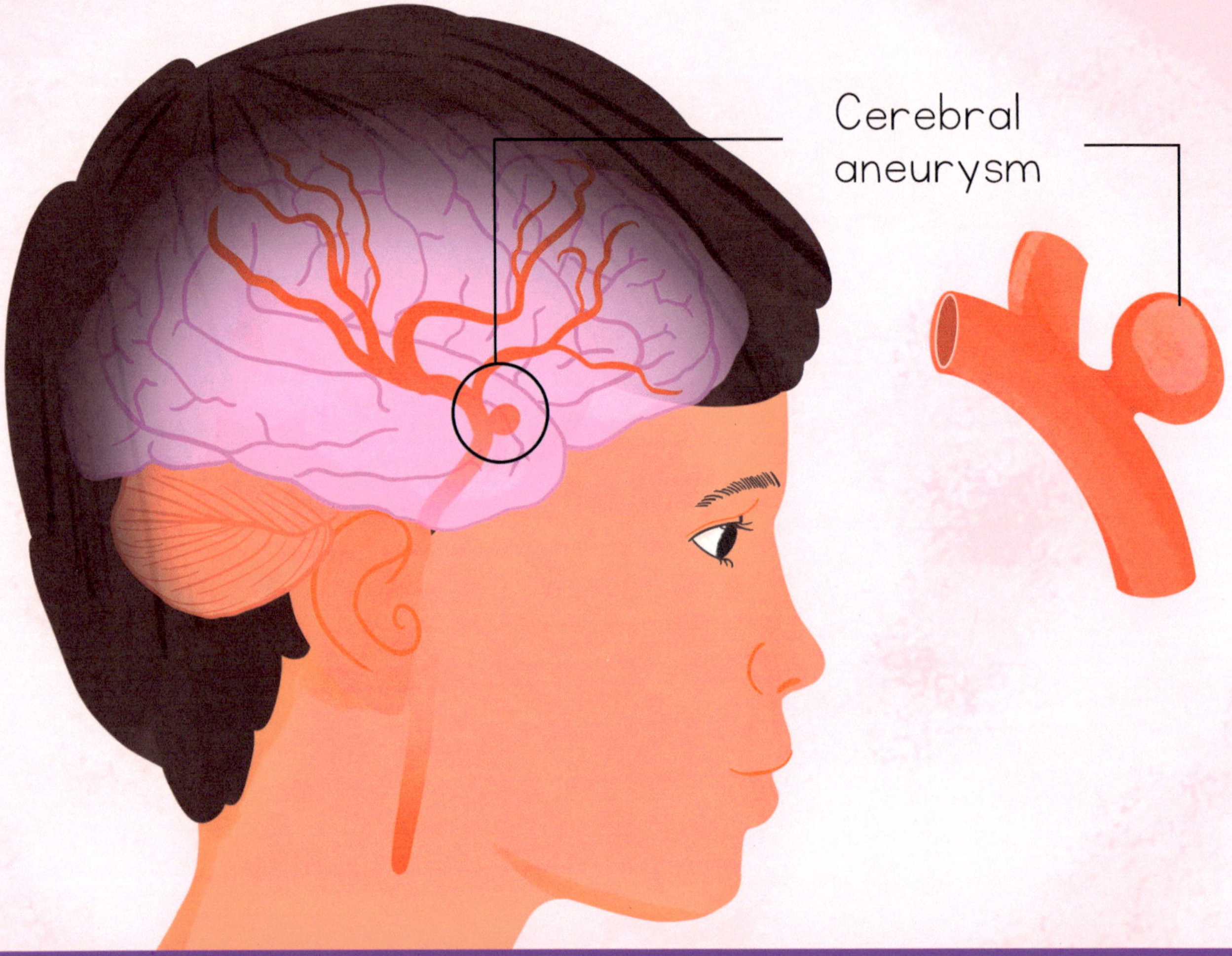

A **cerebral aneurysm** is a ballooning in a weak part of a blood vessel in the brain. If not treated, some cerebral aneurysms can rupture.

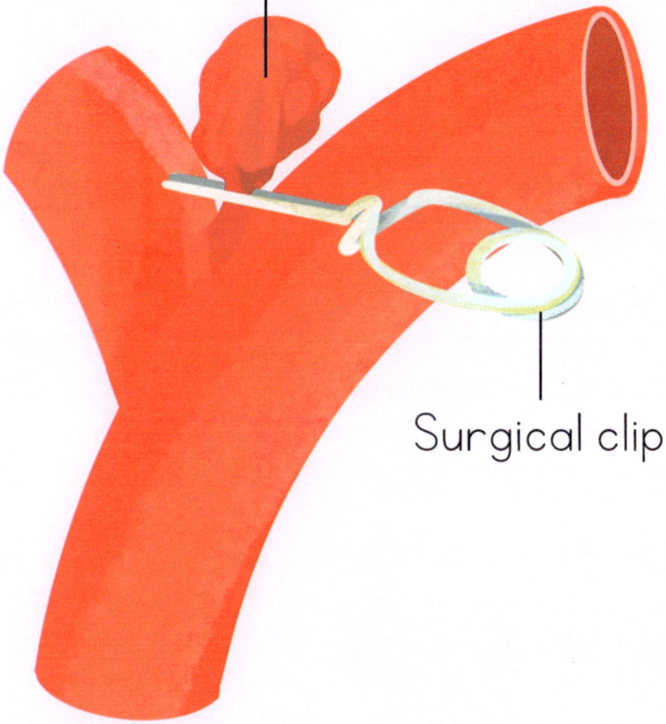

Neurosurgeons can treat a cerebral aneurysm by using a surgical clip to close it off. This is called **surgical clipping**.

Symptoms of movement disorders

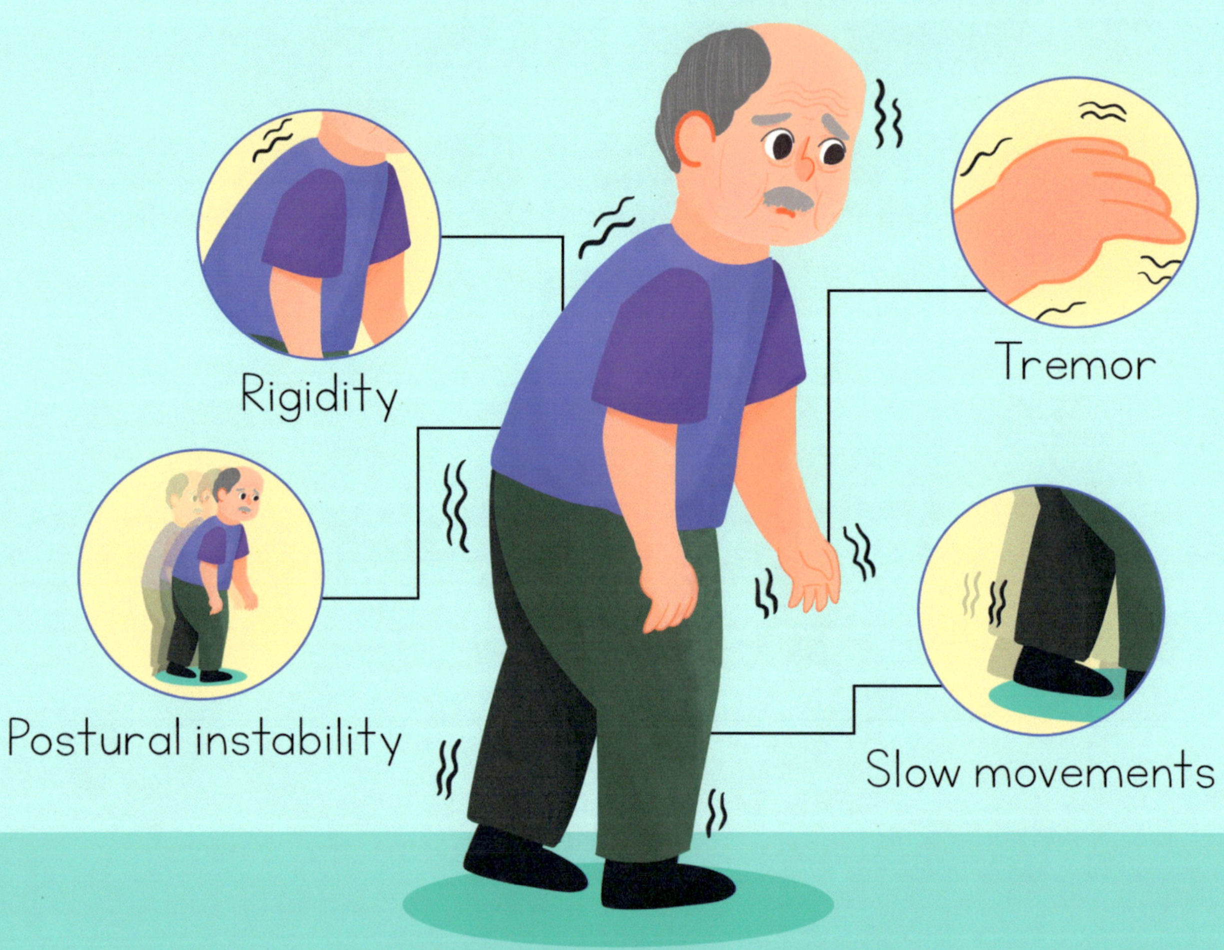

Some people have abnormal movements of the body that they can't control. These are called **movement disorders**.

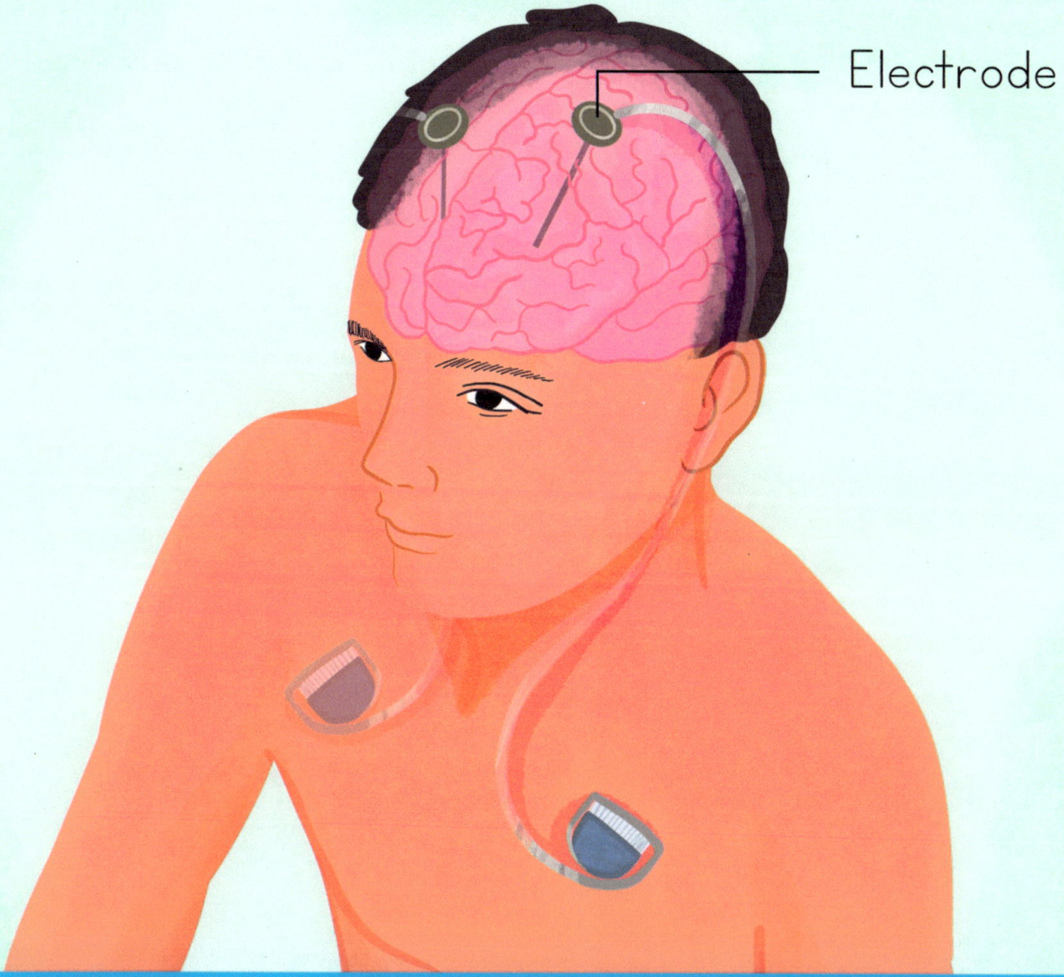

When medications aren't enough, neurosurgeons can place electrodes in the brain to stop the movements. This is called **deep brain stimulation**.

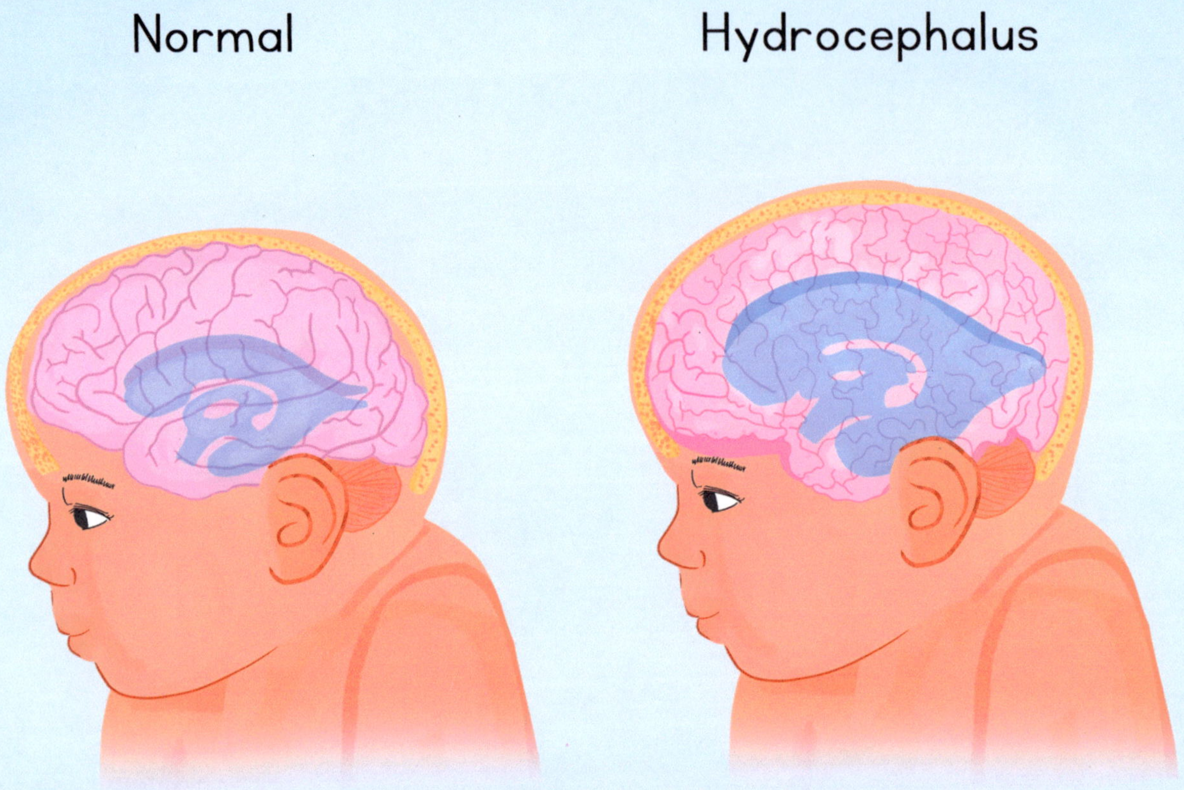

Hydrocephalus is the buildup of cerebrospinal fluid that the brain can't absorb. It can increase pressure and damage brain tissue.

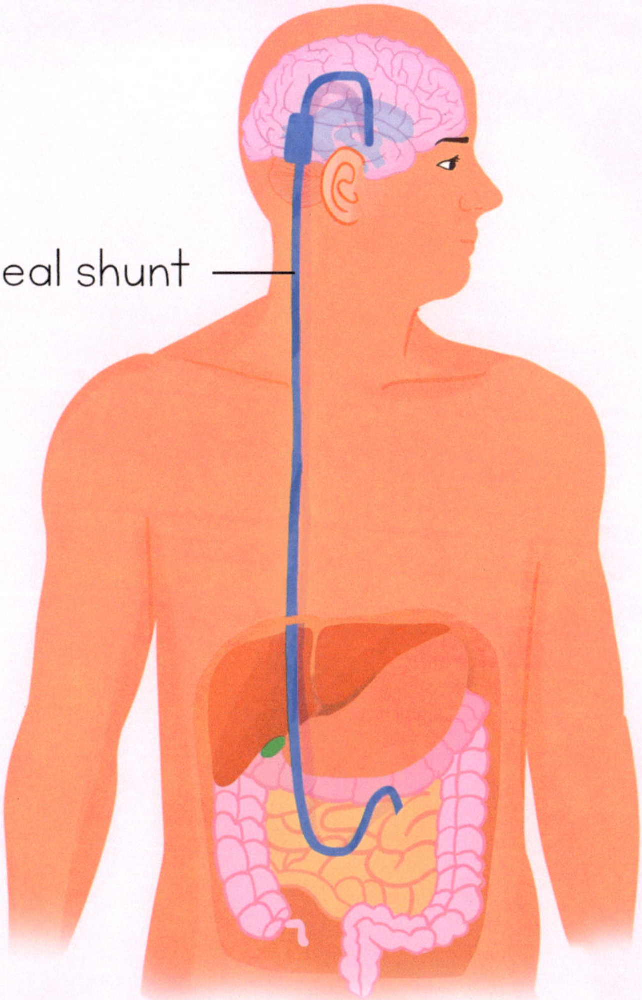

Neurosurgeons can drain this fluid by connecting a silicone tube from inside the brain to the abdomen. This is called a **ventriculoperitoneal shunt**.

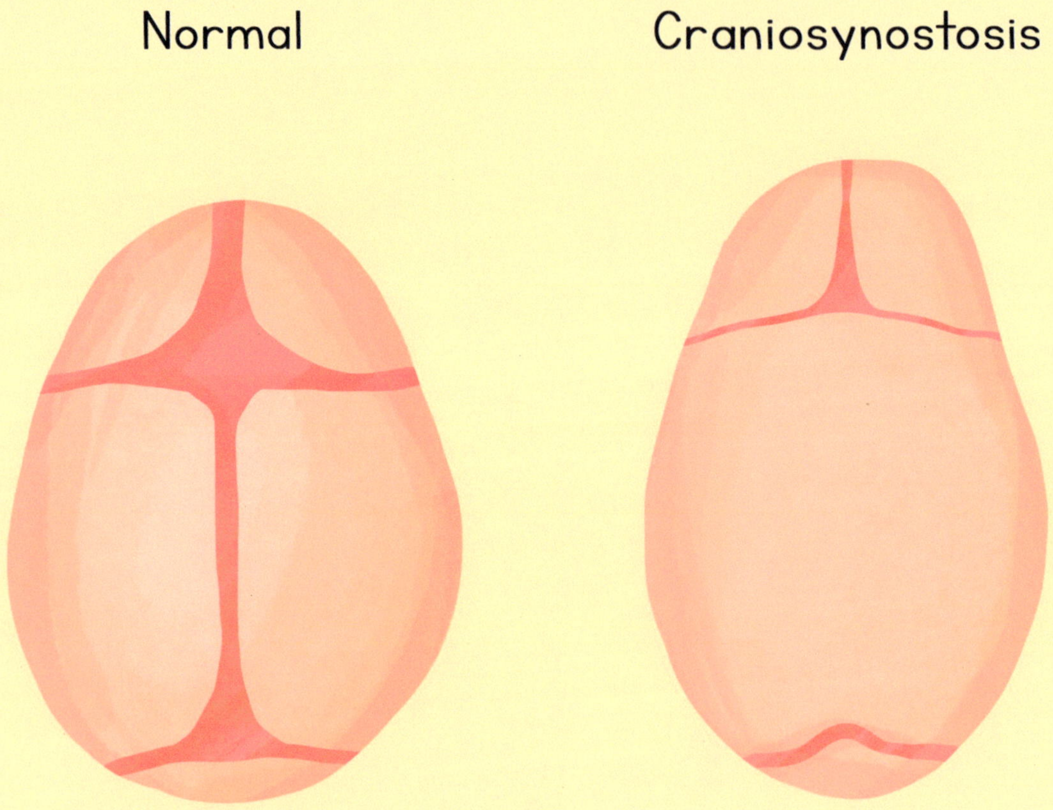

Sometimes, a baby's skull bones fuse too early, causing the skull to have different shapes as the brain grows. This is called **craniosynostosis**.

Cranioplasty

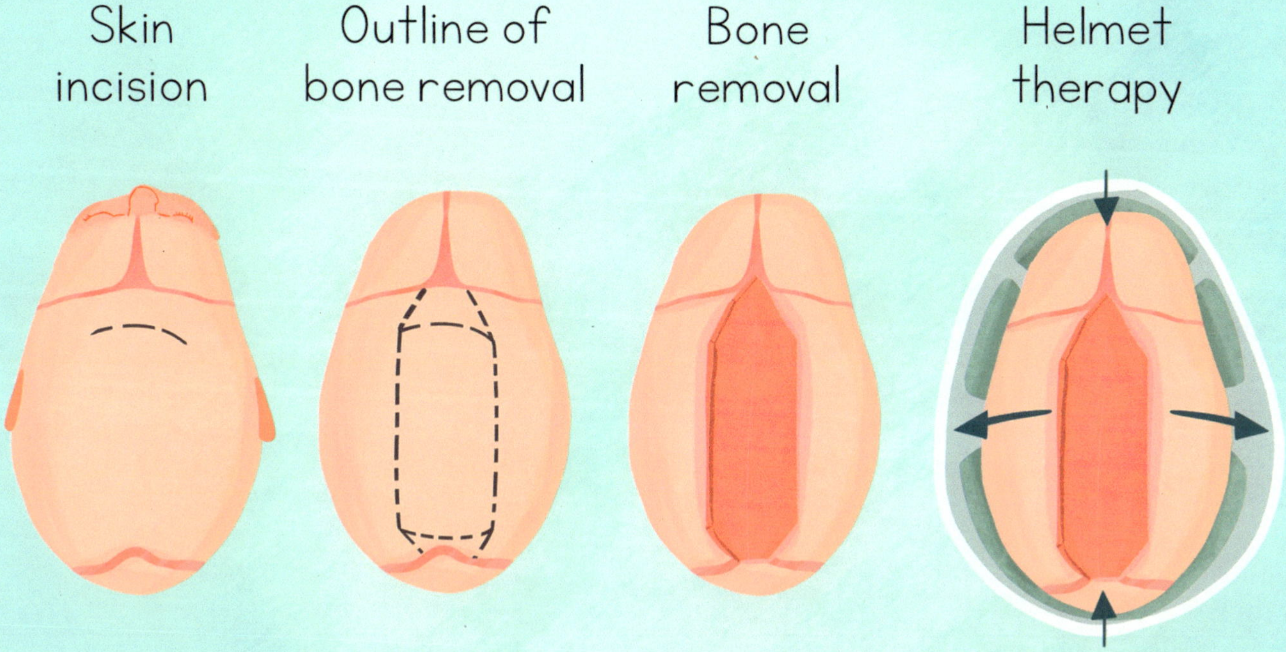

Neurosurgeons can fix these shapes by making special cuts into the bone to remodel the skull. This is called a **cranioplasty**.

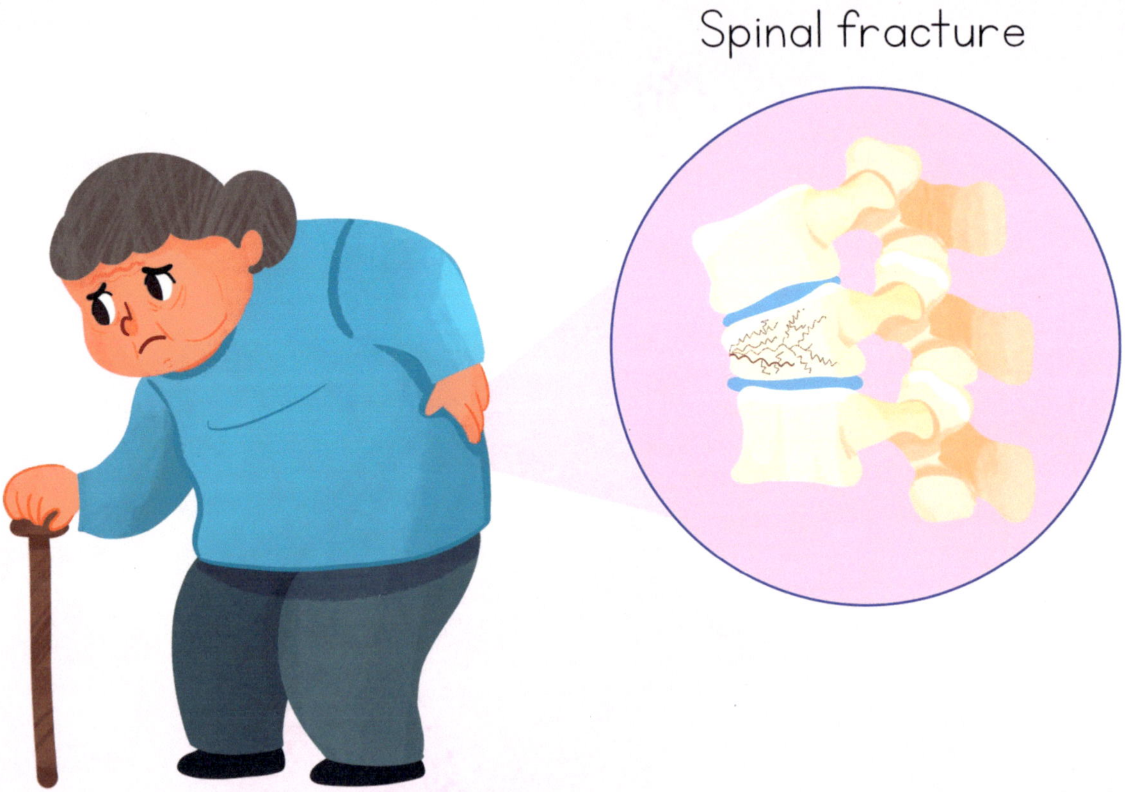

Sometimes, an accident can
break a bone in the spine.
This is called a **spinal fracture**.

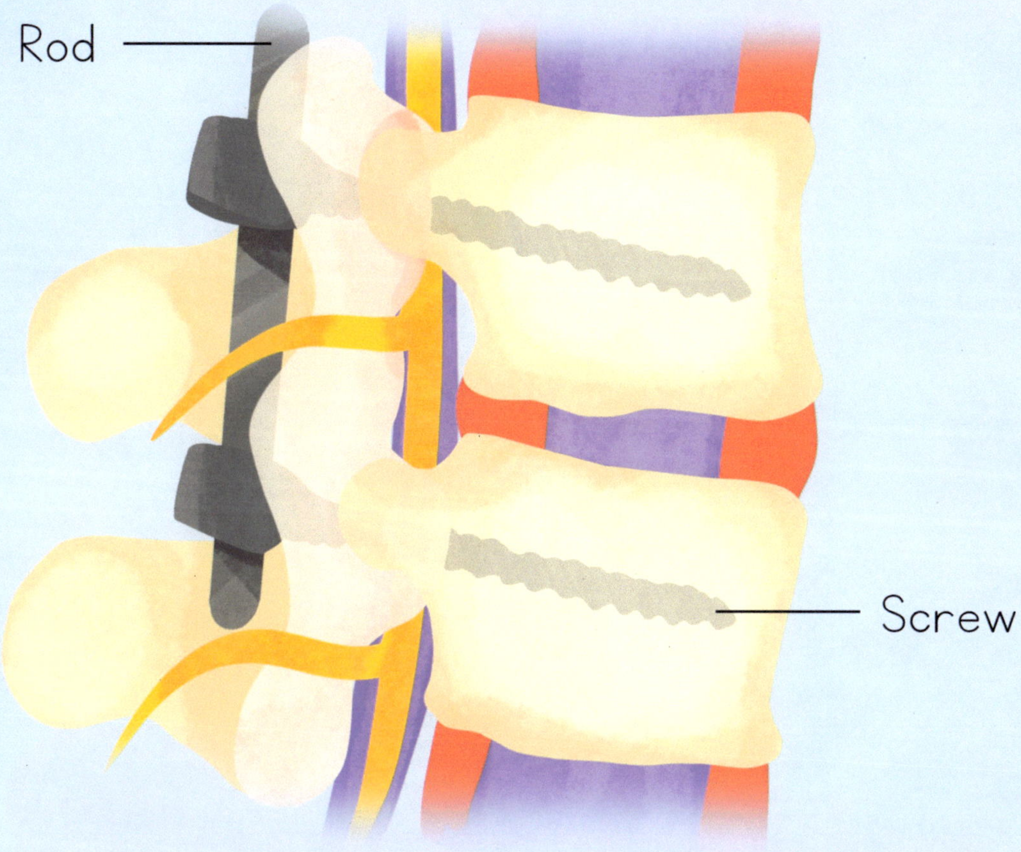

Neurosurgeons can fix this by connecting the bones back to help them heal together. This is called a **spinal fusion**.

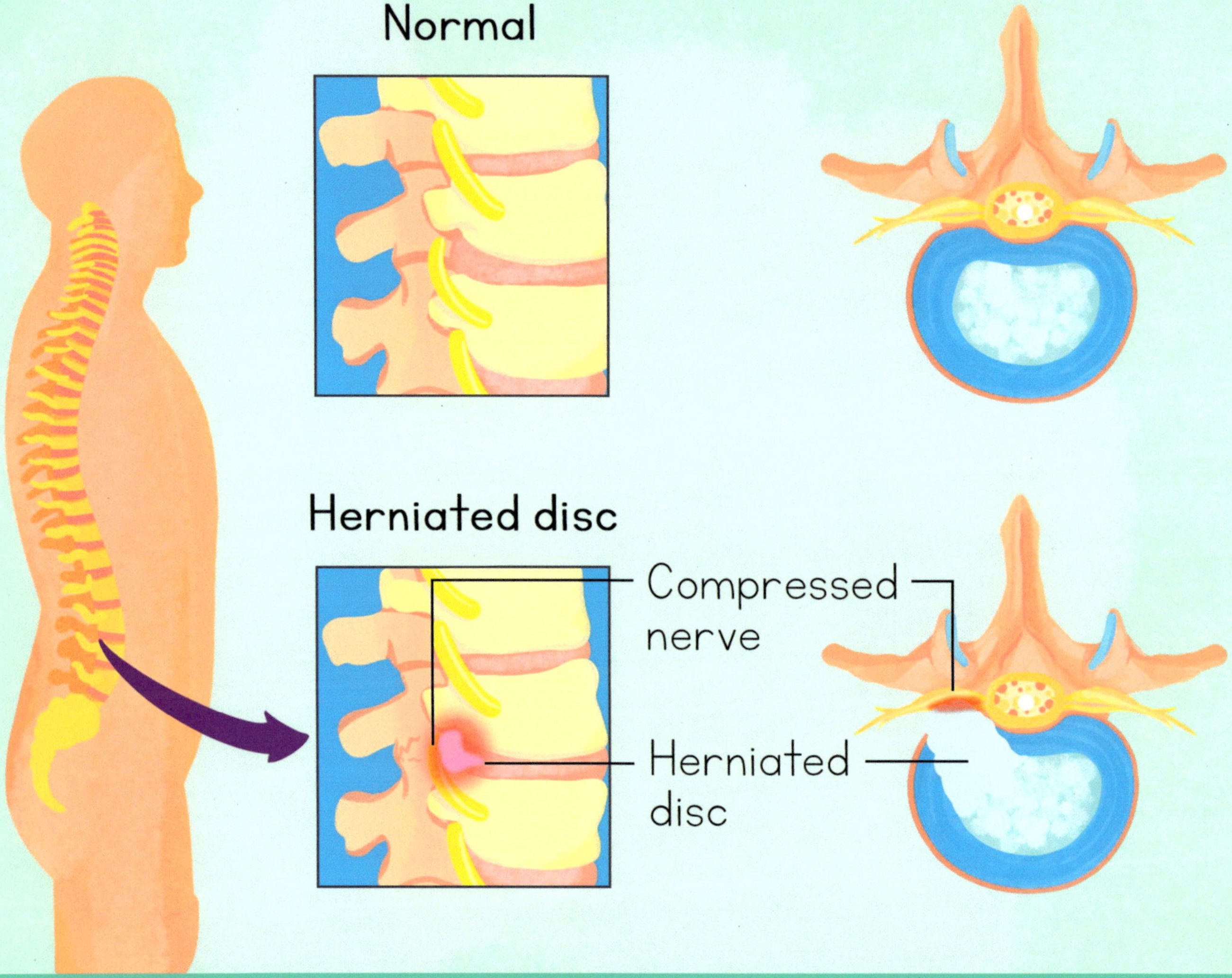

An intervertebral disc can bulge out and compress a nerve from the spinal cord, causing pain, numbness, or weakness. This is called a **herniated disc**.

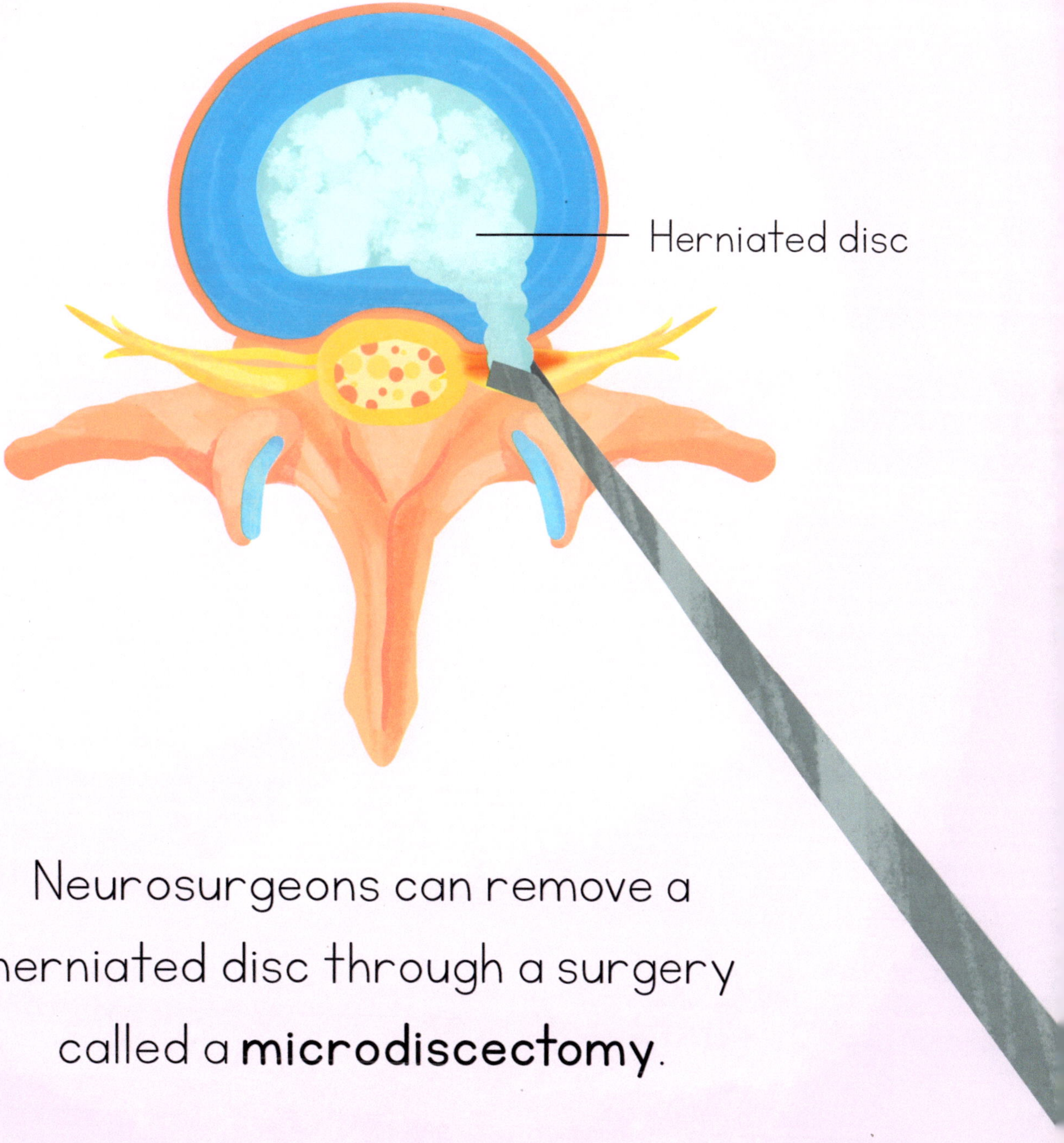

Neurosurgeons can remove a herniated disc through a surgery called a **microdiscectomy**.

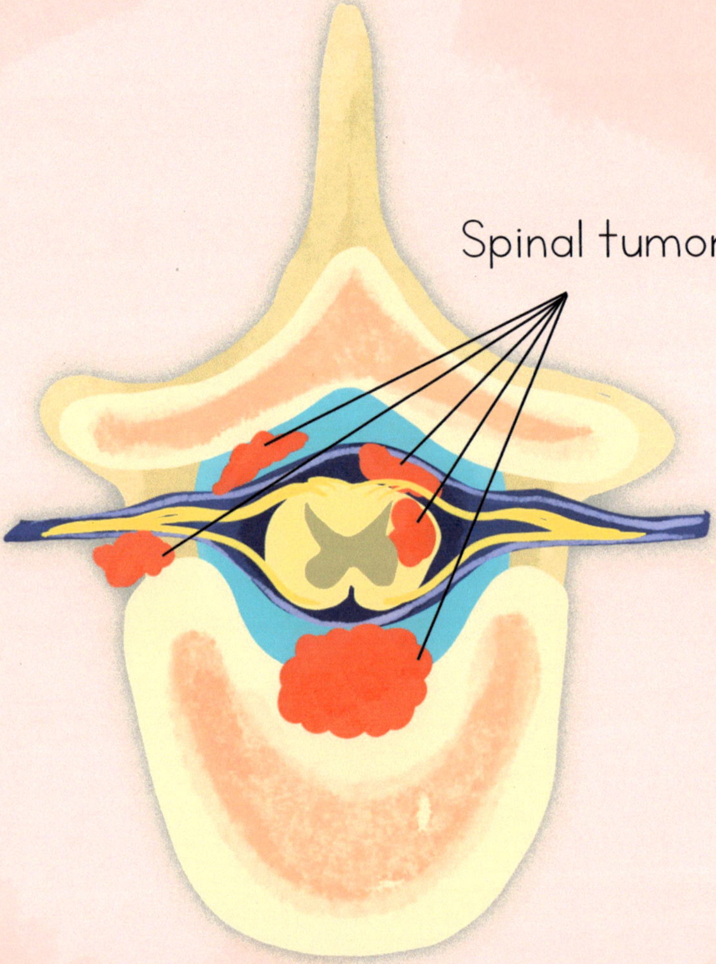

A **spinal tumor** is an abnormal growth of cells in the vertebrae, nerves, or spinal cord. Like brain tumors, there are many types of spinal tumors.

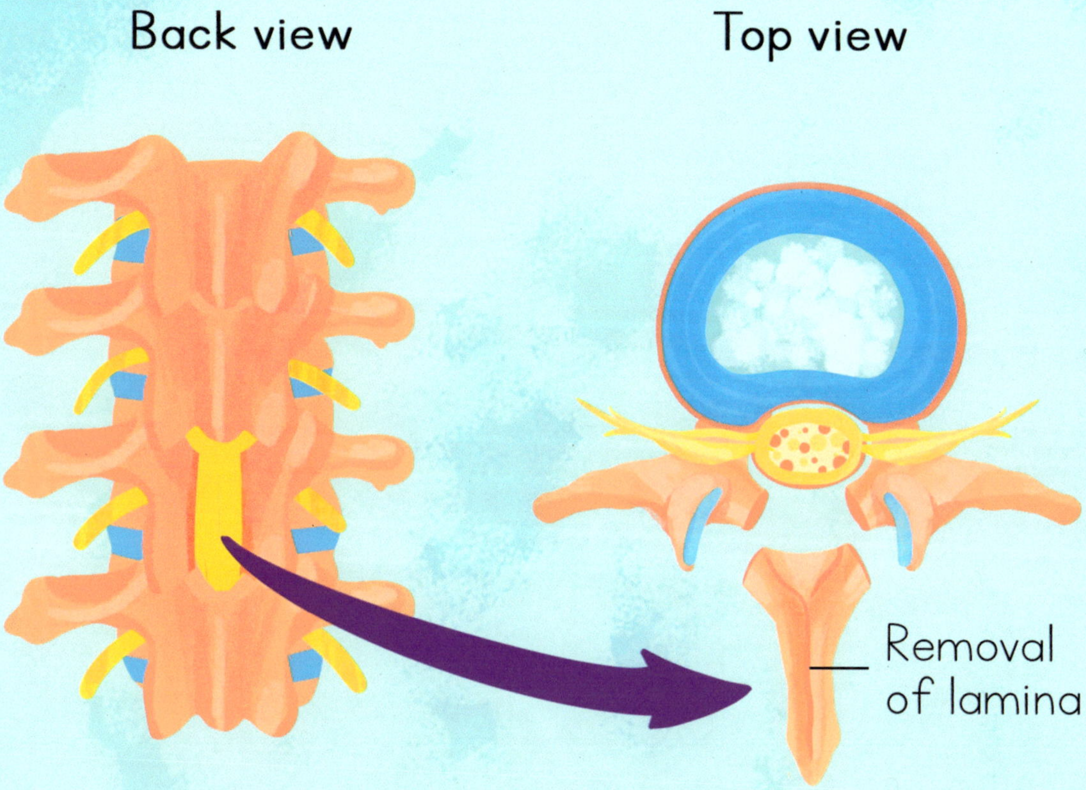

To safely remove these, neurosurgeons remove part of the vertebra, called a **laminectomy**, to access the tumor and take it out.

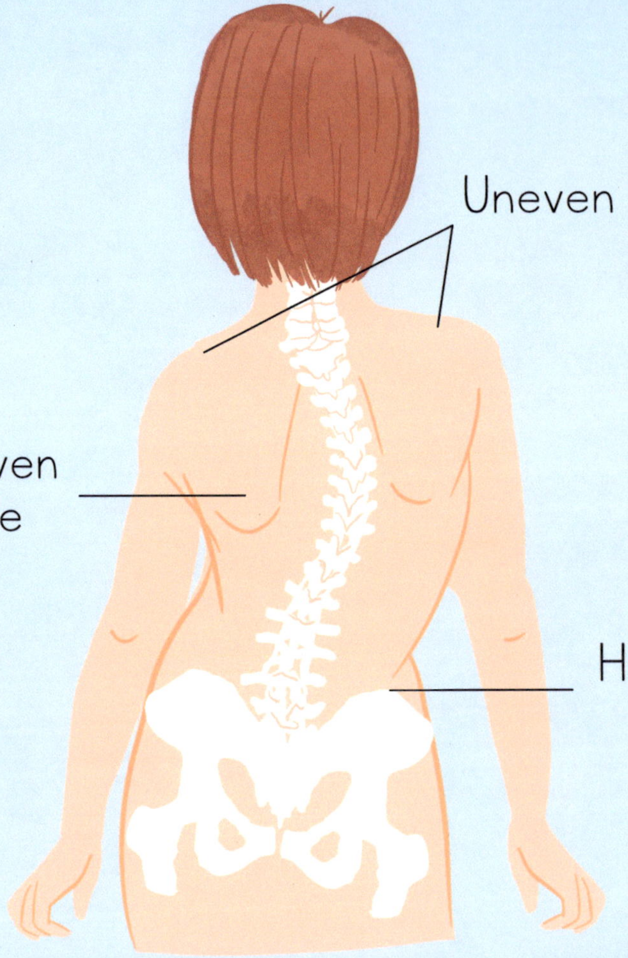

Some people develop curvature of the spine, called **scoliosis**.

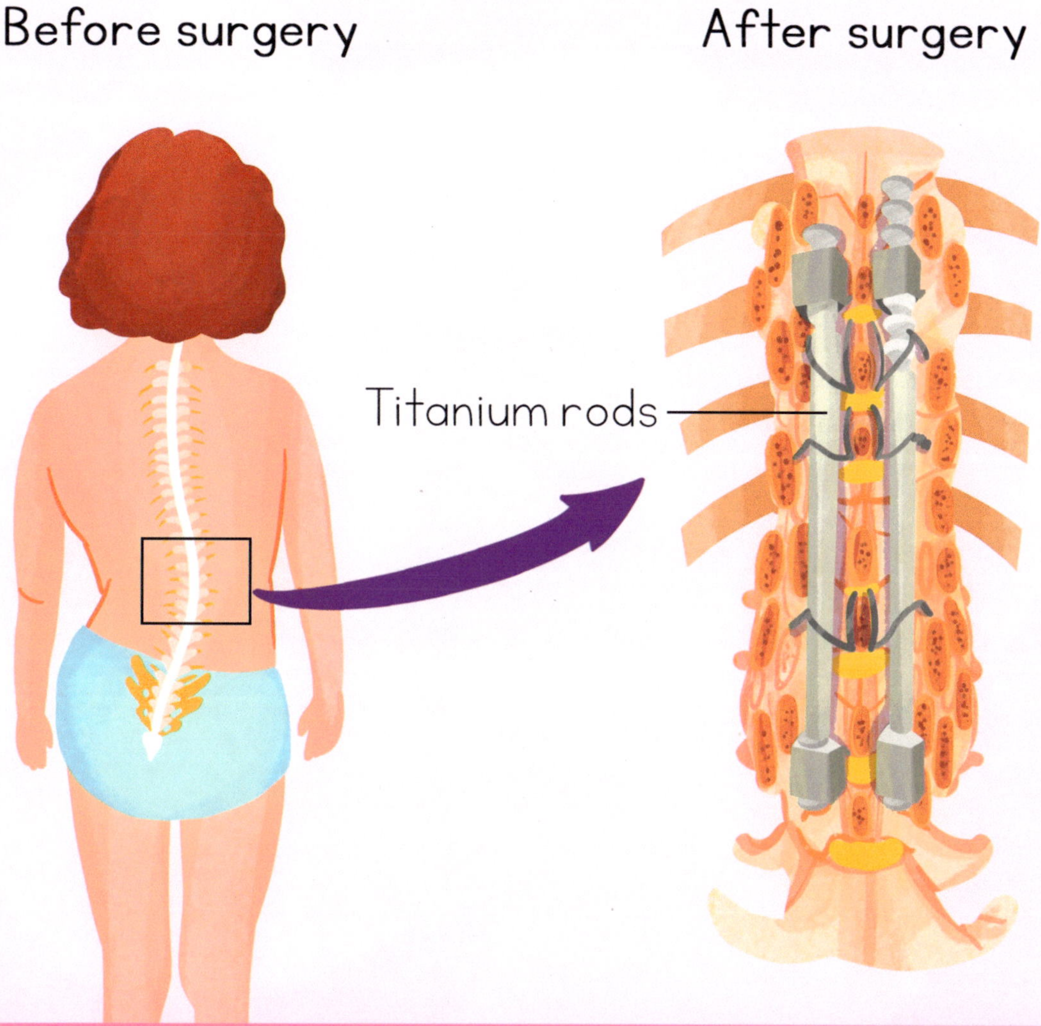

Neurosurgeons can fix scoliosis by using special instrumentation, such as titanium rods and screws, to straighten and support the bones of the spine.

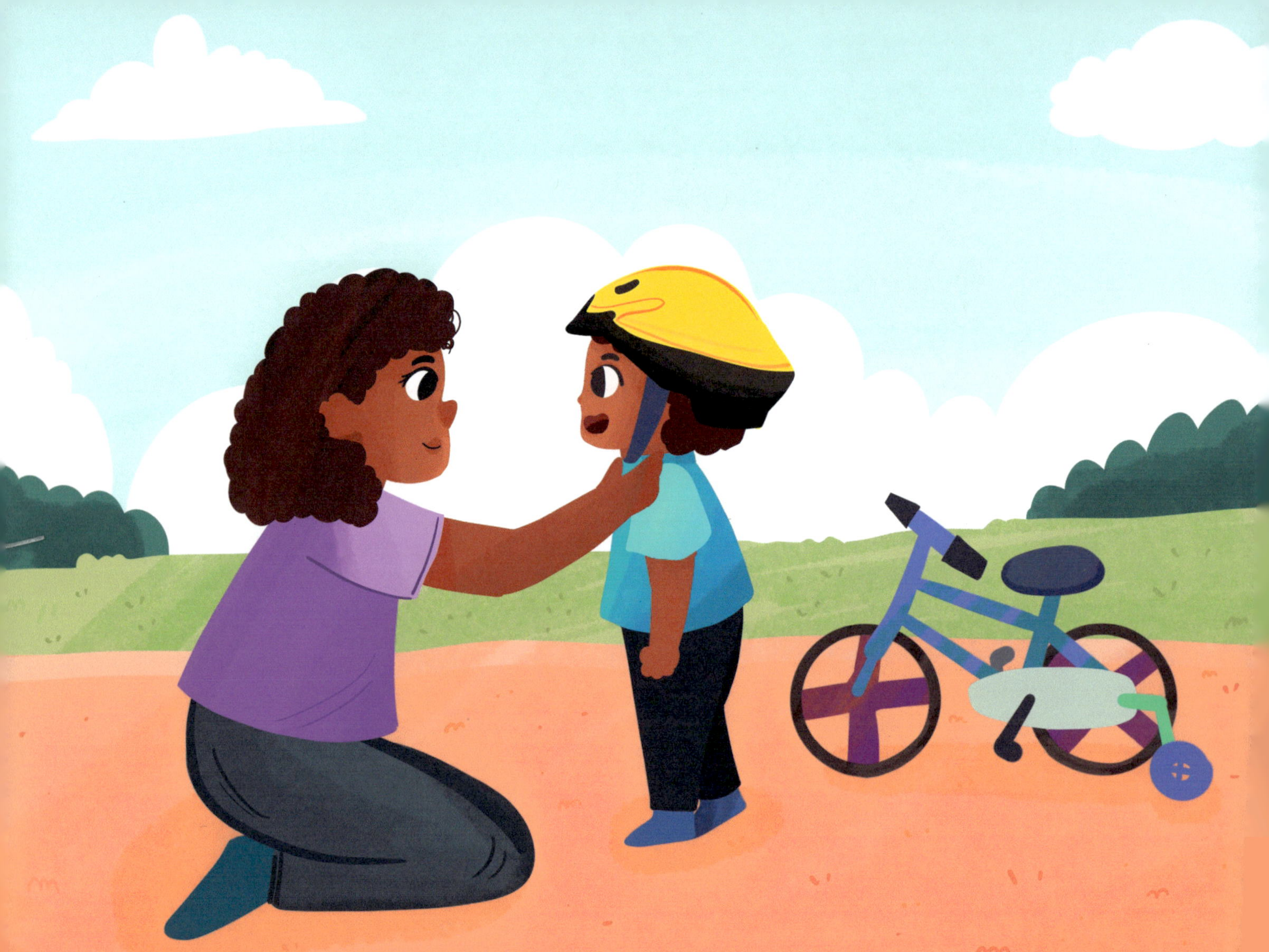

Our brain, spinal cord, and nerves are important organs that play a role in everything we do, so it's very important to protect them from injury.

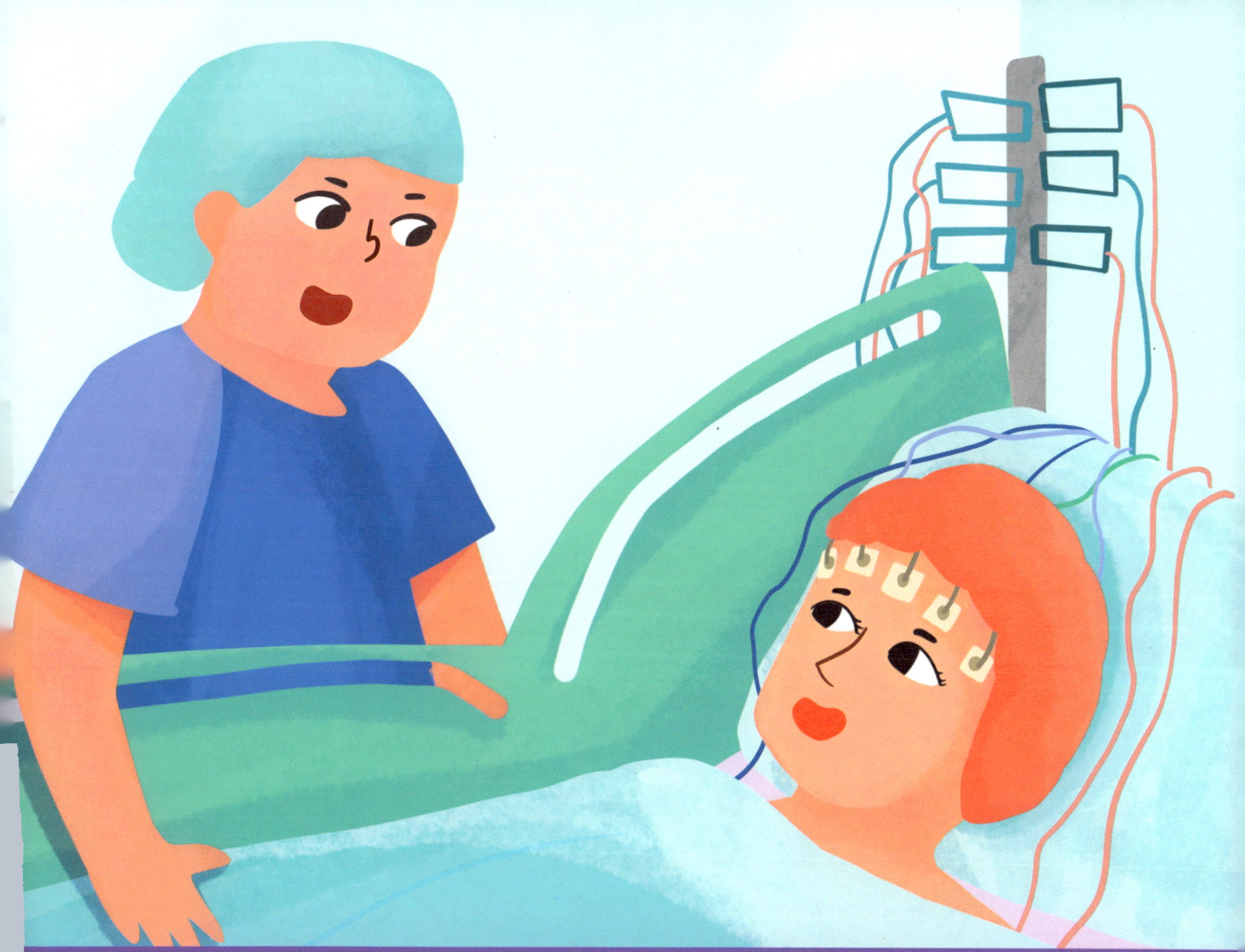

Every day, neurosurgeons help patients with diseases and injuries affecting the brain, spinal cord, and nerves get better.

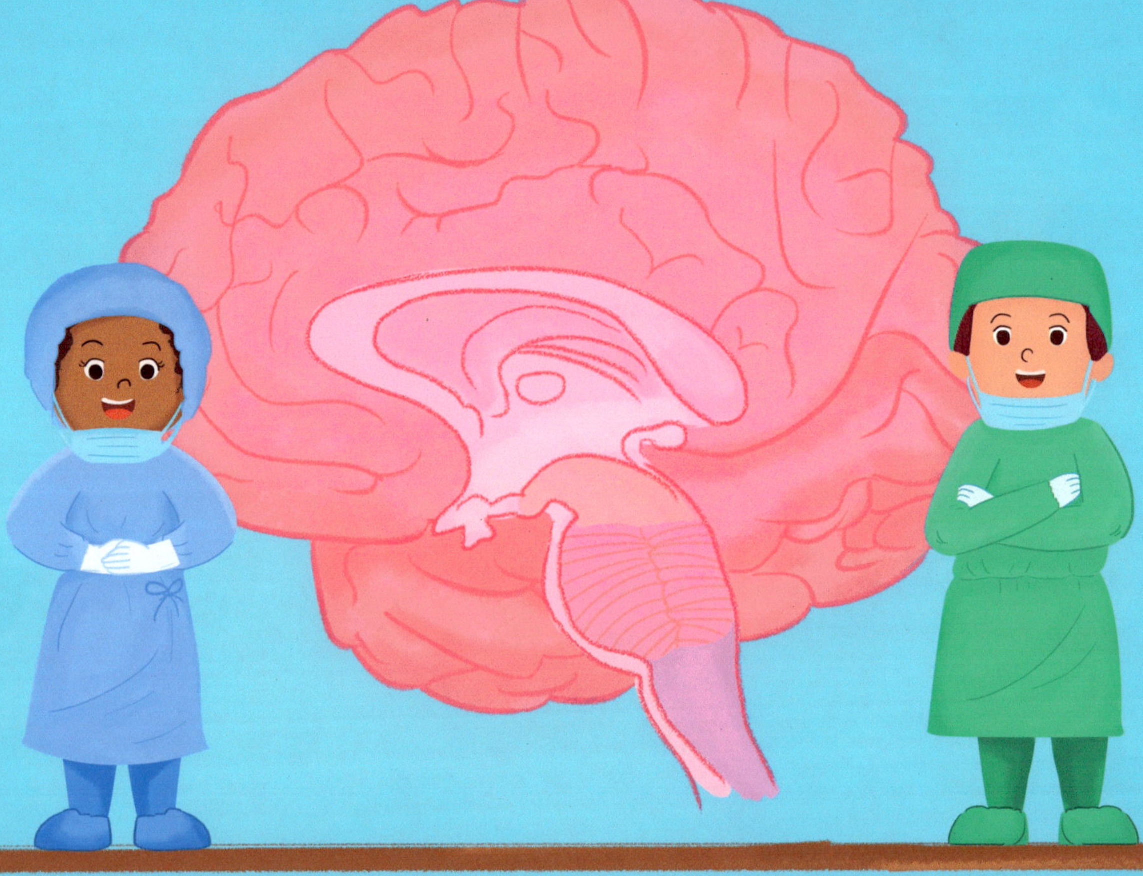

YOU'RE A FUTURE NEUROSURGEON!

Glossary

Brain (brayn): organ within our **skull** that controls all bodily functions; surrounded by a protective fluid called **cerebrospinal fluid**; connects to the rest of our body through our **spinal cord** and **nerves**

Endoscope (EN-duh-skowp): tube-like camera used to look inside the body

Cerebral aneurysm (sr-EE-bruhl A-nyr-i-zm): ballooning in a weak part of a blood vessel in the brain; can be treated by **surgical clipping**

Craniosynostosis (kray-nee-ow-suh-naaz-TOW-suhs): defect in which a baby's skull bones fuse too early; can be treated with a **cranioplasty**

Hydrocephalus (hai-drow-SEH-fuh-luhs): abnormal buildup of fluid in the brain; can be treated with a **ventriculoperitoneal shunt**

Intervertebral disc (uhn-tr-VUR-tee-bruhl): cushion between vertebrae; if bulges out (**herniated disc**), can be treated with a **microdiscectomy**

Intracranial hematoma (in-truh-KRAY-nee-uhl hee-muh-TOW-muh): collection of blood within the skull; can be treated with a **craniotomy**

Movement disorders (MOOV-muhnt duh-SOR-durz): conditions that cause problems with movement; can be treated with **deep brain stimulation**

Operative microscope (AA-pr-uh-tuhv MAI-kruh-skowp): instrument used by neurosurgeons during surgery to make tiny objects look larger

Scoliosis (skow-lee-OW-suhs): abnormal curvature of the **spine**

Tumor (TOO-mr): abnormal growth of cells; can occur in the brain and spine

Vertebrae (VUR-tuh-bray): bones that surround and protect our spinal cord; if broken (**spinal fracture**), can be treated with a **spinal fusion**

Let's review what you learned!

1. What organ in our head allows us to think? What structures protect it?
2. What structures connect our brain to the rest of our body?
3. What are the bones and cushions that make up our spine called?
4. What is a collection of blood in the skull that can be caused by trauma called? If severe enough, what kind of surgery can be used to remove it?
5. What is an abnormal growth of cells in or around the brain called?
6. What instrument can be used to magnify images during surgery?
7. What special camera can be inserted through the nose to help access and remove tumors at the bottom of the skull?
8. What is a ballooning in a weak part of a blood vessel in the brain called? What is one way this can be treated?
9. What are neurologic conditions that cause problems with movement called? When medications aren't enough, how can these conditions be treated?
10. What is the buildup of cerebrospinal fluid that the brain can't absorb called? What can neurosurgeons use to treat this condition?
11. What condition causes a baby's skull bones to fuse too early? How can this be treated?
12. What is the breaking of a vertebra called? How can this be treated?
13. What is a bulging intervertebral disc called? How can this be removed?
14. What is a curvature of the spine called? How can this be treated?

Your Answers

1. ____________________
2. ____________________
3. ____________________
4. ____________________
5. ____________________
6. ____________________
7. ____________________
8. ____________________
9. ____________________
10. ____________________
11. ____________________
12. ____________________
13. ____________________
14. ____________________

Medical School FOR KIDS™

Answer Key

1. Brain; skull and cerebrospinal fluid
2. Spinal cord and nerves
3. Vertebrae and intervertebral discs
4. Intracranial hematoma; craniotomy
5. Brain tumor
6. Operative microscope
7. Endoscope
8. Cerebral aneurysm; surgical clipping
9. Movement disorders; deep brain stimulation
10. Hydrocephalus; ventriculoperitoneal shunt
11. Craniosynostosis; cranioplasty
12. Spinal fracture; spinal fusion
13. Herniated disc; microdiscectomy
14. Scoliosis; special instrumentation, such as titanium rods and screws

Medical School FOR KIDS™

About the Authors

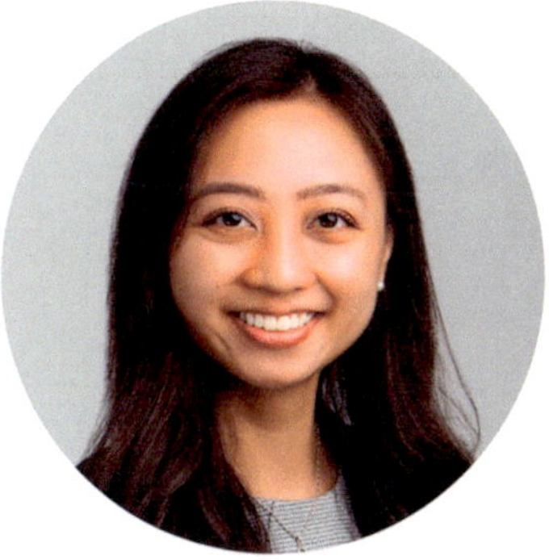

Dr. Betty Nguyen

Betty is a physician specializing in dermatology. She was born in Southern California but spent much of her childhood in Georgia, where she grew up on a chicken farm. Betty studied Biology at UCLA, where she was a Gates Millennium Scholar, and earned her MD from UC Riverside on a full-tuition scholarship. Outside of work, Betty is a certified yoga instructor and licensed scuba diver. She also enjoys journalistic writing and cycling.

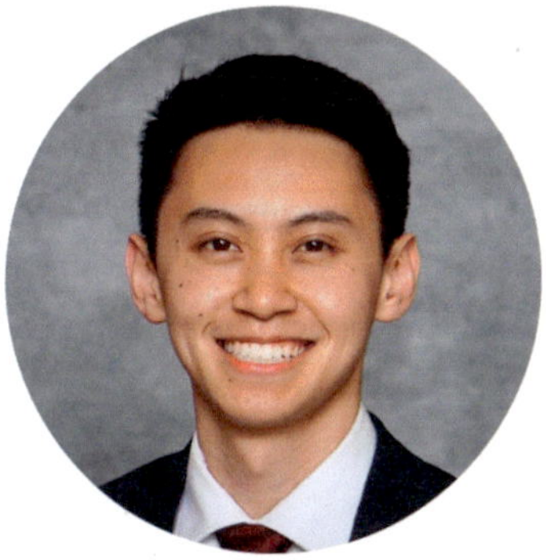

Dr. Brandon Pham

Brandon is a physician specializing in ophthalmology. He was born and raised in Southern California. Brandon studied Microbiology, Immunology, and Molecular Genetics at UCLA, where he was a Barry Goldwater Scholar, and earned his MD from Stanford. He is passionate about medical education for students of all ages. In his free time, Brandon enjoys traveling, playing tennis, and performing card magic tricks.

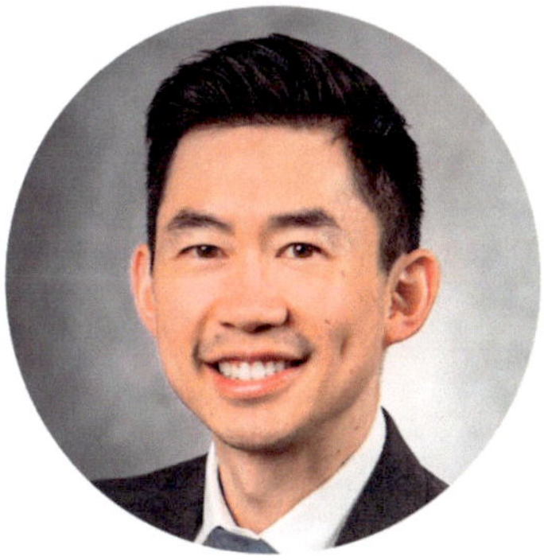

Dr. Martin Pham

Martin is a physician specializing in neurosurgery. He was born and raised in California. Martin studied Molecular, Cellular, and Developmental Biology at UCLA and earned his MD at Northwestern University. He is currently a neurosurgery professor at UCSD, specializing in spinal surgery, and continues to teach and train surgeons. In his free time, he enjoys reading, woodworking, and traveling with his family to show his kids how to live a kind and grateful life.

Check out the rest of the books in our series!

Website: mdforkids.org

Instagram: @md.for.kids

Medical School FOR KIDS™

Made in United States
Troutdale, OR
11/03/2026

56844890R00026